Diets to help
ASTHMA AND HAY FEVER

A concise explanation of the main dietetic rules for successfully treating asthma and hay fever. As well as listing the main types of foods to be avoided the book provides a maintenance diet and stricter diets for the management of acute attacks.

CLEANSING DIET - PAGE 48

ACUTE ASTHM ATTAK - PAGE 57

MEDISINGSFOR —ᴸ - PAGE 73

(ARSENICUM ALBUM 12)

Diets to Help
ASTHMA AND HAY FEVER

R. NEWMAN TURNER
B.Ac., N.D., D.O., M.R.O., M.R.N.

Thorsons
An Imprint of HarperCollins*Publishers*

Thorsons
An Imprint of HarperCollins*Publishers*
77–85 Fulham Palace Road,
Hammersmith, London W6 8JB
1160 Battery Street,
San Francisco, California 94111–1213

First published as *Diets to Help Hay Fever and Asthma* 1970
Second edition published 1989
This edition, revised and updated, 1993
1 3 5 7 9 10 8 6 4 2

© Roger Newman Turner 1970, 1993

Roger Newman Turner asserts the moral right to
be identified as the author of this work

A catalogue record for this book
is available from the British Library

ISBN 0 7225 2911 2

Phototypeset by Harper Phototypesetters Limited,
Northampton, England
Printed in Great Britain by
HarperCollinsManufacturing Glasgow

Contents

Introduction

Asthma and hay fever are such common complaints nowadays that many people accept them as part of their existence. Together with headaches, constipation and a few other ailments they are regarded as something the sufferer has got to 'learn to live with'. Like a rainy or foggy day, they have to be tolerated and most people believe very little can be done about them. If the symptoms become more than just a nuisance and medical advice is sought there is still no satisfaction, for there is no drug or method of treatment in orthodox medicine that can be said to effect a lasting cure for asthma or hay fever.

Possibly one of the reasons for this is the almost total lack of reference to the nutritional aspects of these conditions. But thousands of people have successfully alleviated both hay fever and asthma by the adoption of a sound dietetic regime. For years naturopaths, osteopaths and medical herbalists have helped many sufferers from asthmatic disorders and hay fever by the use of therapeutic diets in conjunction with physical and biochemical readjustment of body functions.

You might feel that you suffer enough already without inflicting the further discipline of a diet upon yourself. But if you hope to cure your complaint, a degree of dietary control is bound to be necessary at some stage and the sooner you start to use a constructive approach the sooner will you begin to feel better. Dietary therapy need not be unpleasant – it is simply a matter of observing certain basic rules and making an interesting menu within the framework of a sound wholefood regime.

This book will show you the principal dietetic rules for the successful management of asthma and hay fever. The main types of food to be avoided, as well as those of which you may need more, are discussed. A maintenance diet, based on the nutritional principles outlined, is given and there are stricter diets for the more intensive treatment of the complaints and management of the acute attacks. The final chapter will give a selection of recipes which contain only those ingredients that would be suitable for your illness.

Our knowledge of dietetics is still very much in its infancy and what information we have is based on clinical experience and a limited amount of research. Our knowledge may, in fact, never be complete, for nutritional requirements vary with every individual, but we know enough to be able to offer hope to the sufferer.

It is the hope of the author that this book will provide the information which will enable you to adopt a more constructive attitude to your health and to enjoy life more fully.

A WORD OF CAUTION

For some individuals with allergic disorders, particularly asthma, an attack may become a potentially life-threatening situation. This can occur in any susceptible individual but is more likely if drugs used to control the condition are withdrawn too rapidly before the body's own coping resources have been sufficiently developed.

The diets recommended in this book are perfectly safe for almost all asthma and hay fever sufferers and, when they bring some relief, you may feel encouraged to reduce the medical treatment or drugs you have been taking. Before doing so, and particularly if you are in any doubt about your ability to undertake such measures, do consult a naturopathic physician or your own doctor for advice.

surprising that the condition is aggravated when there is a disorder of another part of the respiratory system.

Perhaps it is some consolation for hay fever sufferers that their attacks tend to occur only during the spring and summer. At such times pollens, dust, and fungal spores are more abundant and these are allergens – substances which precipitate attacks in sensitive individuals.

HAY FEVER: WHY THE SYMPTOMS OCCUR

What happens is painfully obvious to the sufferer from hay fever. Perhaps more important is why it happens and what can be done about it.

To appreciate the mechanisms involved in attacks of hay fever we must know something of the anatomy and normal functions of the affected area, the nasal passages and sinuses. As you inspire air normally it does not go directly from nasal passage to lungs but circulates through the cavities in the facial bones known as the nasal sinuses. These sinuses are lined with mucous membrane similar to that in the nose. In the hay fever sufferer the mucous membrane is more sensitive than in the normal individual and certain external irritants such as pollens or house dust precipitate an attack. These irritants are called allergens.

ALLERGENS

The susceptibility of hay fever sufferers varies. The majority of people have their attacks in spring and summer, when grass pollens are abundant. In certain areas the condition may continue through the autumn, when plants such as ragweed are in flower. But the condition is not, strictly speaking, just 'hay fever' because other allergens, such as tree pollens, house dust, fungus spores, or animal hair, can precipitate an attack.

The reason that these allergens cause such severe irritation and subsequent symptoms is believed to be because they are composed of protein molecules which are larger than those of normal proteins which we absorb from our food. Healthy blood vessels and mucous membranes have a fine, closely-knit structure which only allows smaller molecules to penetrate. In individuals showing an allergic reaction, however, the poorer quality of the blood vessel walls and membranes permits the entry of the larger protein molecules which act as irritants.

The irritant action of these allergens causes the release from the tissues of a substance called histamine which brings about swelling of mucous membranes. Sometimes the swelling is more widespread once the allergen has entered the blood-stream and the eyes and face become puffy. In severe attacks even the extremities, such as the nose and ears, may be affected.

Tests to discover specific allergens, followed by a course of injections to desensitize the individual, seldom have any lasting benefit. Anti-histamines are widely used, but

13

they do no more than alleviate the symptoms of congestion in hay fever. They merely antagonize what is a normal defensive reaction by the body and do nothing to correct the underlying imbalance which has resulted in the release of the histamine in the tissues.

Nasal sprays and inhalants are not, of course, considered a cure, and their repeated use can also have a permanently damaging effect on the nasal mucous membranes.

ASTHMA

Asthma is characterized by paroxysmal attacks of shortness of breath with wheezing due to narrowing of the bronchi and distension of the air sacs. Air is trapped in the distended air sacs and the patient is unable to breathe out properly. It is therefore impossible for much fresh air to be taken into the lungs and, as the spasm becomes worse, the neck and shoulder muscles are brought into play in an attempt to make the fullest possible use of the limited lung capacity.

The severe attack will generally have to be broken by the use of a relaxant drug but these become less effective as time goes on unless constructive measures are taken to overcome the complaint and remove the cause. When this is done it is possible to reduce the frequency and severity of attacks and remove the dependence on drugs.

The tendency to asthma is inherited and it is generally regarded as being an allergic condition, that is, attacks are usually precipitated by substances such as pollen, house dust, or animal hair, to which the sufferer is sensitive.

In naturopathy we do not attach so much importance to the allergy as to the underlying cause – the factors which have rendered the individual more sensitive to the allergens which precipitate the attack.

Allergens apart, there are basically two factors that can trigger attacks of asthma: emotional stress and catarrhal infections.

Nervous Asthma

This usually develops after an emotional experience. Most frequently in young children the first attack can be traced back to the birth of a younger brother or sister, or to the mother's absence through illness for a period of time. Subsequent attacks may be precipitated by any emotional upheaval or challenge, such as impending exams. The attack is characterized by a dryish wheeze and breathing difficulty and there will be some coughing due to accumulation of mucus because of the spasm in the lungs.

Catarrhal Asthma

The onset of catarrhal asthma usually follows a bad cold or an attack of bronchitis in infancy. The accumulation of mucus in the lungs causes congestion and subsequent respiratory embarrassment. If there is a heredity tendency to asthma subsequent colds will always carry the risk of chest involvement with an asthmatic attack developing, particularly if antibiotics or other 'cold cures' are used.

TREATING THE WHOLE PERSON

It should be obvious from the foregoing descriptions of the mechanisms of asthmatic disorders and hay fever that constructive therapy is required to increase the resistance of the affected areas and reduce their sensitivity, as well as measures to improve the general health of the sufferer. By tackling the overall condition of the patient and not just treating his local symptoms, a great deal of progress can be achieved, progress of a lasting nature.

One of the most important aspects of these conditions is the nutritional one.

CHAPTER TWO

How and Why Diet Can Help

The previous chapter explained the physiological changes that occur in asthma and hay fever. Sufferers from these complaints are so often told that diet will make no difference to their condition. This is untrue, as the food we eat affects the functions of our body considerably. It provides us with energy and materials for growth and repair of tissue and after these requirements have been met there is a residue of waste which must be eliminated.

In normal health a balance is maintained between assimilation of nutrients and elimination of impurities. This balance can become disturbed and in the presence of a hereditary weakness, or various other factors, ailments such as asthma and hay fever can develop.

Corrective nutrition is one of the ways of treating the cause of these complaints and by following a balanced dietary programme you will be achieving far more than by the continual use of preparations which give only temporary relief of the symptoms.

Symptomatic relief is, of course, often necessary, but it is both useless and harmful if it is relied upon to the exclusion of constructive measures to correct the disordered metabolism which has given rise to the condition.

There are three ways in which one's diet can affect asthma and hay fever:

1 By **excess** of foods which can act as irritants, or have a toxic effect resulting in production of more catarrh. Such food items as milk and starches fall in this category. Their harmful effect may be very small but the cumulative action, when taken regularly over a long period, may contribute to the development of the symptoms.

2 By **deficiency** of various vitamins, minerals and trace elements. This may come about by eating refined foods such as white flour, white sugar and canned or frozen foods, from which much of the nutritional quality has been removed or lost. The regular intake of such foods will result in a deterioration in the tone of the mucous membrane and a general lack of resistance.

3 By an **allergic reaction**. Certain foods may cause an allergic reaction, part of which may be the symptoms of hay fever. Included in this category are strawberries and shell fish. These foods can only cause an allergic reaction in the individual who is particularly sensitive to them.

Foods do not normally precipitate attacks of asthma but there are some isolated examples which will trigger off an attack in susceptible individuals at a time when they are otherwise in good health.

Some people can develop what may be termed an allergy to quite ordinary foods simply by taking excessive amounts of such foods over a number of years. In these cases the respiratory or other symptoms develop not because the patient is allergic but because the body is trying to eliminate the excess mucus and to restore the balance that is necessary for the normal functions of the respiratory organs.

Such items really fall into the first category of dietary excesses. Allergy to other substances such as dust, animal hair and pollens can often be overcome by increasing the natural resistance and toning the mucous membranes by the application of sound nutritional principles and the use of homoeopathic or herbal medication.

WHAT YOU CAN DO

If you want to overcome your asthma and hay fever it can be done with a determined effort to correct dietary errors and by adopting a nutritional regime which will maintain a high level of health.

It is advisable to start by cutting out or reducing all those foods which have a harmful effect in one way or another. Then you should ensure that the diet is well balanced, with adequate proportions of the foods which are particularly necessary to increase resistance and general health against asthma and hay fever.

At some stage, depending on the severity and on how long you have suffered from the complaint, it may be wise to follow a stricter diet, or even carry out short fasts, in order to speed up recovery. This may be necessary in any case when there is an acute attack, for the system is better able to overcome the symptoms when less energy is being used for digestion and it can be made available for the eliminative effort. Instructions on the various stages of dietary treatment are given in the chapters which follow.

CHANGE FOR THE BETTER?

When you change your diet there will usually be an improvement in your general well-being and a gradual reduction in the symptoms of your asthma or hay fever. Don't be disappointed, though, if, after a few days or weeks, you experience a slight aggravation of symptoms. These may take the form of a bit more wheeziness, nasal discharge, or a cold, and even other symptoms which you might not associate with your respiratory system. Both asthma and hay fever sufferers, for example, may have a history of skin disorders, especially childhood eczema, and in the process of getting better again may experience some dryness or irritation of the skin at vulnerable sites. Other transitory symptoms which can occur include diarrhoea and headaches.

All these are quite reasonable responses by your system at it begins to gain the vitality necessary to throw off an old toxic burden. Colds and other acute symptoms are the body's way of doing this and should not be suppressed with antibiotics or other drugs. If you feel better in general, even though some symptoms are undergoing temporary aggravation, you can be reasonably sure that they are no more than that. If you are in doubt about how to handle the situation, however, consult a naturopath who will be able to recommend safe ways of helping you through what is termed the 'healing crisis'.

Once you get over this, perhaps aided by herbal, homoeopathic, or acupuncture treatment – all of which can assist in appropriate cases – you will continue to make gradual progress. Lasting recovery can take several years to achieve, but, with perseverance, you can gain much more control over your own health.

A BASIC ESSENTIAL

The adoption of a dietary plan is a basic essential in the treatment of both asthma and hay fever and without doing this there is little hope of permanent recovery. Diet alone, however, will not be sufficient in the majority of cases. The balancing of organ function and vitality by acupuncture will certainly be of benefit, or you may require a herbal or homoeopathic prescription, to correct body chemistry and improve the tone of the tissues. Even psychological factors should be considered, as both asthma and hay fever can frequently be the physical expression of some emotional stress or anxiety.

If you take any drugs for asthma or hay fever no attempt should be made to reduce the dosage unless you have the guidance of a naturopath. The drugs may have suppressed the symptoms and helped to alleviate the acute attacks but if they are stopped suddenly there may be an aggravation and an eliminative reaction which is too great for the vitality to respond to. It is better to await the gradual improvement that will come with a better diet and to reduce drug amounts or frequency of dosage step by step, substituting a herbal or homoeopathic support if necessary.

CHAPTER THREE

Some Foods You Should Avoid

As mentioned earlier some foods can have an adverse effect upon health by their cumulative action, creating imbalance and deficiency. A direct relationship between the intake of these foods and the onset of asthma or hay fever has not yet been proved, but their effect in lowering general health and resistance is quite definite.

Some food items may be taken for many years without apparent adverse effects but it is the gradual build up in the system of certain of their constituents to a level at which they disturb the normal functions of certain organs that is important.

The body attempts to neutralize and eliminate any harmful substances that are ingested with our food and symptoms may not become apparent until the burden becomes too great, or there is some disturbance of eliminative functions. These dietary factors, super-imposed on constitutional or structural weaknesses, can precipitate your illness.

Listed in this chapter are some of the more obvious trouble-makers in the average diet which should be avoided altogether, and some of which whose intake you should considerably reduce. This does not mean that there will be little left in the diet worth enjoying, for in succeeding chapters we shall consider foods which may be taken and indeed some which are essential to maintain health.

MILK AND CERTAIN MILK PRODUCTS

When the cells of the membranes lining the nasal cavities and sinuses are irritated by foreign bodies they secrete mucus as a protective mechanism. Similarly, when an allergen causes the release of histamine in the tissues, and the consequent swelling, mucus is again produced. When mucus production becomes excessive, catarrh is formed. Catarrh consists of protein and carbohydrate and the more foods of that nature taken in the diet, the greater will be the tendency to catarrhal secretions.

Milk consists of protein, fat, and carbohydrate, in almost equal proportions, and, whilst it is frequently regarded as a complete food, it does not seem to be very well assimilated by many people after infancy. This is chiefly because the ratio of the proteins and fats in cow's milk is such that it is more difficult to digest than other foods. Furthermore, many adults have insufficient lactase, the enzyme that helps us to digest milk products containing the sugar lactose. The result of a high intake of milk and milk products, such as cheese, is more catarrhal secretion.

LACTASE IS NEEDED TO DIGEST MILK PRODUCTS.

MUCUS IS BODY'S PROTECTIVE MECHANISM

Milk, and the harder varieties of cheese, should, therefore, be eliminated from your diet if you are an asthma or hay fever sufferer. In hay fever this may not remove the cause, but it goes some way towards alleviating the symptoms by reducing the catarrhal secretion.

Yogurt should also be avoided in the early stages of your treatment and during any acute attacks, although this may be included in a balanced diet at a later stage.

Foods made with milk, such as milk puddings, custards, and blancmanges, and drinks such as cocoa or coffee with milk, should be avoided. A small amount of milk may be taken in tea, provided you do not drink large quantities of tea. In drinks such as tea, or other beverages, it is preferable to use a low-fat milk substitute such as soya milk, which is obtainable from health food stores.

Low-fat cheeses are permitted and a good quality cottage cheese or ricotta cheese are better than the harder varieties, and are easier to digest.

One further argument against milk as a food is that some individuals have been found to be allergic to it. This is not a common allergy but it may exist in a mild form without being very obvious to the sufferer. Sometimes the antibiotics administered to cattle are passed through to the consumer in milk and in many cases this has been thought to be responsible for the development of certain conditions.

FATS AND FRIED FOODS

Animal fats in the average diet occur chiefly in milk and its derivatives which have already been referred to. They

CAN HAVE LOW FAT CHEESE
& COTTAGE CHEESE.

have a high content of saturated fatty-acids and as such they are more difficult to digest than vegetable oils, which are rich in the type of unsaturated fatty-acids which we require to maintain health. The less efficient our fat digestion is, the more likelihood there is of developing gall-bladder disease. The liver and gall-bladder must be functioning at an optimum level if general health and resistance are to be maintained. You should, therefore, reduce the amount of animal fats in your diet and use instead the vegetable oils, such as sunflowerseed oil.

The frying of foods also renders the fats less digestible, and this method of cooking is to be avoided in the early stages of your treatment.

SUGAR   WORST OFFENDER!

Sugar, especially refined white sugar, comes high on the list of forbidden foods. While you are treating asthma and hay fever you should not take even brown sugar, or sugar substitutes.

Sugar is a highly concentrated food which contributes to a wide variety of complaints. It not only acts as an internal irritant to the mucous membranes, but also tends to leach the body's calcium reserves and in this way lowers the general resistance. There is definite evidence to suggest that those who take large amounts of sugar in various forms actually create a chronic state of low blood-sugar level. Low blood-sugar means less vitality and poor resistance to disease. Individuals with a tendency to low blood-sugar levels are more inclined to be allergic and

"EATS" CALCIUM - MUCUS FORMING.

many have high histamine levels.

Foods which contain sugar must also be avoided or reduced in quantity. Cakes, biscuits, proprietary puddings, canned fruit and, of course, sweets and chocolates, all contain added sugar (or artificial sweeteners, which have much the same effect) and these must be eliminated from the diet.

Natural sugar, which is better assimilated, and provides all the body's energy requirements, may be taken in the form of honey, dried fruits, and grapes. These contain minerals and trace elements which are required in our diet whereas refined sugar does not. A good quality honey should always be used when a sweetener is required. Some authorities suggest that honey is of specific benefit in cases of asthma and hay fever, but this would not be suitable if you suffer from low blood-sugar.

HONEY NOT SUITABLE FOR PEOPLE WITH
LOW BLOOD SUGAR.

STARCHES

The same restriction applies to the starchy foods as to sugar. All starches are reduced to sugar during digestion and, if the intake is excessive, their ultimate effect is similar.

Bread, especially that made with white flour, pastry, cakes, biscuits and bananas should be reduced or even avoided altogether. Moderate amounts of wholemeal bread, or brown rye biscuits, or pumpernickel, are permitted, except when on a strict eliminative diet. As a general rule any starchy food in the diet should be in the minor proportion.

COFFEE DISTURBS LIVER & GOLD BLADDER FUNCTIONS. (causes mucus)

STIMULANTS

Under this heading come such items as coffee, strong tea, alcohol, tobacco and spices. Whilst no direct cause or relationship has been established between, say, coffee drinking and asthma or hay fever, the caffeine present in the beverage does have an adverse effect on general health, disturbing, in particular, the function of the liver and gall-bladder. The liver is responsible for the breakdown of all impurities in our food to a form which can be eliminated. When there is disturbance of liver function, the level of toxic substances in the blood rises and there is, consequently, a greater burden upon the mucous linings of the sinus and nasal cavities.

You would, therefore, be wise to avoid drinking coffee regularly. Use instead a decaffeinated coffee, or better still a coffee substitute or other beverage, which can be obtained from a health food store.

The same restriction applies to tea, to a lesser degree, and to alcohol which also has a high sugar content. China tea is better in general than the Indian variety.

Table salt should not be used, either as a condiment or in cooking. Salt tends to cause fluid retention in the tissues. Prolonged cooking of vegetables in salt also causes a loss of many of the vitamins and minerals naturally present. The only type of salt permitted, for cooking if necessary or at the table, is sea salt, obtainable from a health food store.

SALT CAUSES FLUID RETENTION.

USE ONLY SEA SALT!

MEAT AND FISH

It is not the purpose of this book to advocate vegetarianism, although this is undoubtedly a healthier type of diet for the majority of people. Meat is not well digested and causes a high level of impurities in the system, and if you are not already a vegetarian it is certainly advisable to reduce the amount of meat that is eaten.

For many people, however, it would be unwise to make a sudden change to a vegetarian diet as this may create problems of readjustment. As the asthma and hay fever sufferer should reduce the intake of the dairy proteins, some meat and fish may be desirable as an alternative to these, although there are many nutritious vegetarian alternatives available nowadays.

Whatever meat is eaten should be of the lean varieties. Fish is preferable as this provides a higher content of vitamins A and D, and is generally more readily digested.

CHAPTER FOUR

Some Foods You Require

Most of the foods referred to in the previous chapter can be avoided altogether, or reduced considerably, and the stricter one is about this the greater will be the improvement in health. There are, however, many foods which you must include in a balanced diet to maintain a high level of health and resistance to disease.

Such foods should be rich in their content of vitamins, minerals and trace elements, and one way of ensuring this is to eat foods as near their natural state as possible. Always try to select foods which have been grown naturally, without the use of artificial fertilizers and chemical pesticides.

The best way of ensuring that your food has been naturally grown and prepared with the minimum loss of nutritional value is to shop at a health food store. The produce available there is selected because it has not undergone the considerable refinement, and removal of nutrients found in the natural state, that is the case with many mass-produced foodstuffs nowadays. Some of the larger supermarket chains also stock organically grown produce.

VITAMINS "A" + "C" = ASTHA VITAMIN

Diets to help ASTHMA AND HAY FEVER

The two most important vitamins required by sufferers from asthma and hay fever are vitamins A and C.

VITAMIN A

Vitamin A is found chiefly in the form of carotene, a precursor of the vitamin, present in vegetables and some dairy foods, such as eggs. Carotene is fat-soluble, which means that a sufficiency of unsaturated fatty-acids must be available for it to be converted into vitamin A in our bodies. It is, therefore, necessary to use vegetable oils, such as corn oil, or sunflower-seed oil. Adequate supplies of vitamin A are essential to the health of skin, hair and mucous membranes, and to increase resistance to infection.

EAT CARROTS TO MAINTAIN HEALTHY MUCUOUS MEMBRANS

Carotene Content of Vegetables and Fruits

Carrots, mature	20,000 I.U. per 100g
Spinach	13,000
Carrots, young	10,000
Cress	8,000
Watercress	5,000
Apricot	2,000
Lettuce	2,000
Tomato	1,200
Brussels sprouts	700
Cabbage	500

VEG. OILS ARE NEEDED TO CONVERT CAROTENE TO VITAMIN "A".

The adequate utilization of vitamin C also depends on the presence of vitamin A. Vitamin C is important to increase resistance to infection, and it also has an anti-allergic reaction. It is, therefore, necessary in abundance in the diet of hay fever sufferers.

TAKE VITAMIN "C" AGAINST ALLERGIES!

Food Sources of Vitamin C

FRUITS

Apples	4.60 mg per 100g
Blackberries, raw	21.00
Grapefruit	40.00
Guava	300.0
Melon	32.00
Orange	49.30
Strawberries	60.00
Raspberries	24.00
Blackcurrants	57.00

VEGETABLES

Cabbage	78.00 mg per 100g
French beans	14.00
Tomato, raw	23.00
Watercress, raw	80.00

FRUIT AND VEGETABLES

From the above it will be seen that these should form the greater proportion of the diet, and, preferably, they should be taken in the raw state. Almost any type of fruit or vegetable may be eaten, except some soft fruits to which you may be allergic. Bananas should be avoided, however, because of their high starch content.

Vegetables and fruit provide nourishment and energy with little or no toxic effect upon the system. They are rich in many of the vitamins and minerals we require, particularly vitamins A and C which are essential for the natural functions of the mucous membranes.

Fruits also provide natural sugar for energy. Dried fruits are particularly valuable in this respect and should be included in the diet in place of sugar and other sweeteners.

It is important to ensure that your daily menu contains a generous proportion of some of those fruits or vegetables mentioned, which are rich sources of vitamins A and C.

PROTEINS

Although it is important to avoid the excessive intake of certain types of protein these are, none the less, an important part of the balanced diet. They are essential to provide heat and energy for the body, and the best forms in which to take them are the vegetable proteins, such as the pulses, cereal grains and nuts.

You should, therefore, use such vegetables as beans, peas, lentils and soya products. The cereal grains, such as millet, buckwheat and brown rice may be used as these also have a relatively high protein content.

Nuts are an excellent source of protein, and with few

exceptions, nut kernels contain between 12 per cent and 15 per cent. (It is also worth noting that walnuts have a vitamin C content which compares very favourably with other sources, such as orange juice or rose-hip syrup.) Nuts should, therefore, be included in the balanced diet and may form the basis of savoury dishes, or be ground and sprinkled over fruit or other desserts.

Sunflower, pumpkin, and sesame seeds are also convenient sources of protein as well as providing essential fatty acids, needed to carry fat-soluble vitamins and to counteract inflammation.

CARBOHYDRATES

Carbohydrates are also necessary as energy foods. The vegetable carbohydrates should form the greater proportion of the diet. Any cereals in the diet should be of the whole grain type, such as millet, buckwheat, rice, couscous and whole wheat. NO.

CHAPTER FIVE

The Basic Diets

If you are not accustomed to what is known as a food reform diet and the nutritional approach to asthma and hay fever is new to you, you may find it difficult to make a complete change immediately. The transition from a conventional diet to a healthier, more balanced one is best made gradually.

The adjustment by the body to a rapid change in eating habits may often precipitate some unpleasant minor symptoms, which are relatively harmless in themselves and may, indeed, be an indication that the body is responding by the elimination of toxic encumbrances. Normally they should be allowed to take their course, but if in doubt you should obtain the professional advice of a naturopath or medical herbalist.

The basic diets will serve as a transition towards the stricter diets that may be necessary for the treatment of these conditions, details of which are given in the chapter which follows, but if you only suffer mildly from either asthma or hay fever, a change to the basic diet may be all that is required to achieve a considerable improvement.

If the conditions are more severe, then it may be essential to undergo the stricter diets.

Severe attacks will have to be treated with the usual symptomatic measures but if the severity or frequency of the attacks increases you should obtain professional advice.

Try to eat as much food as possible in the raw state, and you should always endeavour to start a meal with some raw fruit or salad. When cooking vegetables or fruit, do it only long enough to make the food tender. They should be cooked for a short time in only a small quantity of water, without salt being added. This minimizes the loss of essential vitamins and minerals.

BASIC DIET FOR HAY FEVER SUFFERERS

On Rising

Drink of freshly extracted orange, pineapple or apple juice, or warm water with lemon juice and honey. If fresh extraction of juices is not possible use bottled or canned, pure unsweetened juices obtainable from a health food store or high-class grocer.

Breakfast

For those who take very little breakfast, or none at all, but like to have something to drink, the following are recommended:

Pure fruit juices or vegetable juices as above, or a special drink (see page 88), weak China tea with lemon or a little milk (a soya-milk or similar substitute are recommended, but a small amount of cow's milk in tea is permitted at this stage), a cereal beverage or coffee substitute.

To eat, choose from the following, according to appetite:

Whole nuts with raisins.

Soaked, dried apricots or prunes, or other dried fruits as available.

Fresh fruit, or fruit salad made from apples, pears, grapes, oranges, peaches, plums, melon, etc., as available.

Puréed or grated apple, with wheatgerm and raisins.

Stewed or baked apple with wheatgerm or raisins.

A home-made muesli (see p.88) or porridge served with soya milk.

A small portion of pure goat's or sheep's milk yogurt may be taken with any of these dishes at breakfast.

Two or three slices brown rye biscuit, pumpernickel, or wholemeal toast, with a little butter or sunflower oil margarine, and savoury spread or honey.

Mid-morning

Warm drinks: coffee substitute, weak tea, or savoury drink, e.g. a yeast extract beverage – one teaspoonful in a cup of hot water.

Cold drinks: pure fruit or vegetable juice.

Do not eat.

Mid-day Meal

Small glass of freshly extracted vegetable juice as an apéritif, or a serving of single or mixed vegetable soup.

Large or small combination salad, according to appetite. A portion of cheese or milled nuts or dried fruit may be taken with the salad, or you may have a serving of a savoury, such as a millet or nut dish, or a potato baked in its jacket with a little vegetable oil. One or two slices of pumpernickel, or rye bread, or wholemeal bread may be taken, with a little butter or sunflower oil margarine and a savoury spread, if desired, with the salad.

Dessert
Fresh or dried fruit, using only honey or maple syrup for sweetening, if required. Fruit jelly. Carrageen (seaweed) mould. Egg custard. Muesli.

Milled nuts or wheatgerm may be added to a fruit or vegetable salad.

Afternoon

Drinks as for mid-morning. It is preferable not to eat, but if you are accustomed to having something, one or two wholemeal biscuits or some fresh fruit may be taken.

Evening Meal

Fruit or vegetable juice apéritif, or vegetable soup (if not already taken at lunchtime).

Savoury dish with one or two conservatively cooked vegetables. Mixed vegetable stew. Combination salad as at mid-day meal.

Dessert
Fresh or dried fruit or fruit jelly as a mid-day meal.

On Retiring

Drink of fruit or vegetable juice, or warm drink of cereal beverage made with water and a little milk substitute, or other drink as desired.

Do not eat.

BASIC DIET FOR ASTHMA SUFFERERS

On Rising

Fresh fruit juice; or hot water, lemon juice and honey; or weak tea.

Breakfast

Selection of fresh fruit as appetite demands; or muesli with fresh fruit and goats' milk yogurt, or soaked dried fruits, e.g. apricots, prunes. Baked or stewed apple with raisins and wheatgerm. 1 or 2 slices wholemeal toast, brown rye biscuit with a little butter or vegetable oil margarine and savoury spread or honey.

Between Meals

Fresh fruit juice, e.g., apple, pineapple, grape, orange juice. If fresh juice is not obtainable, the unsweetened bottled or canned juices from a health food store or high-class grocer are permitted. Some juices such as the orange, pineapple and concentrated apple may require dilution with water. Weak China tea or dandelion coffee or coffee-substitute. Certain savoury spreads may also be dissolved in hot water as a drink. (Always use the low-salt type of spread.)

Lunch

Large combination salad consisting of a selection of the following vegetables according to availability: lettuce, cabbage, watercress, cress, endive, chicory, carrots, celery, cucumber, beetroot, tomatoes, and onions or garlic. The coarser ingredients should be grated or chopped finely. Add cottage or other low-fat cheese, raisins, or fresh fruit to flavour. Milled nuts or wheatgerm may be sprinkled on top. Use a home made dressing if desired. 1 or 2 slices of wholemeal bread, or rye bread or a biscuit with a little butter or vegetable oil margarine. A potato baked in its jacket may be eaten with the salad.

For dessert, fresh or dried fruit dish or a little cheese and biscuits or natural fruit jelly, baked egg custard, carrageen jelly, or soya-based desserts.

Afternoon

Drink as recommended above. If food is desired a wholemeal biscuit or some fruit and nuts may be taken.

Evening Meal

<u>Aperitif of freshly extracted carrot or beetroot juice</u>, or a pure bottled vegetable juice available from health food stores. As an alternative, vegetable soup, flavoured if necessary with a savoury spread or yeast extract, may be taken.

<u>Savoury dish made with various protein foods such as eggs, meat, fish, pulses, nuts, or cereal grains</u>. Two or three conservatively cooked vegetables. Potatoes, boiled or baked in their jackets, <u>millet, or brown rice may be taken with the main dish and vegetables</u>, if they do not already contain much pastry or other cereal.

<u>For dessert, take fresh fruit salad, or soaked dried fruit</u>, or any dish made with fruit. <u>Sprinkle milled nuts, or wheatgerm, or pine kernels over the fruit salad and add a little maple syrup or honey to sweeten if desired</u>. As an alternative dessert a fruit or carrageen jelly may be taken.

On Retiring

A warm fruit or savoury drink may be taken, or if preferred, a little fresh fruit. Avoid any starchy or milky food or drink at this time of day.

NOTE
The mid-day and evening meals may be transposed if desired, or you may have a combination salad at both

meals instead of a warm dish. It is preferable to have one salad meal per day. If it is difficult to have this type of menu for your mid-day meal while you are at work, you should either take fresh fruit, or sandwiches made with wholemeal bread or biscuits, or have the cooked meal at mid-day and the salad meal in the evening.

CHAPTER SIX

Advanced Diet Programmes

When you have followed the balanced diet for some weeks, you may feel able to undertake a short, stricter diet to increase elimination. This more advanced phase of treatment will bring greater benefits to your health and further relief from the symptoms of asthma and hay fever.

These more specific dietary measures are certainly necessary if you suffer from any aggravation of the symptoms, which may occur after you have been on the balanced diet for some time. This aggravation can be regarded as an encouraging sign – an indication that a greater eliminative effort is being made by the body.

People in whom the conditions have been long-standing, or are particularly severe, may find it necessary to repeat the strict diet a number of times. If there is not a definite improvement when this is done, however, do not lose hope, for chronic conditions require 'chronic treatment' and it may well take several years of perseverance during which time your complaint will become gradually less severe and troublesome.

The sufferer from asthma which is predominantly

nervous in origin would be well advised not to undertake stricter diets without the guidance of a practitioner. By following the basic diet the nervous asthma sufferer will effect sufficient improvement in the physical components of his condition, and manipulation and relaxation techniques will be necessary forms of treatment to follow up with.

There are two types of strict diet for both asthma and hay fever; the short-term and the long-term. The longer strict diet gives a greater eliminative stimulus to the body, but it is not wise to undertake it without the advice and guidance of a naturopathic practitioner unless you are accustomed to food reform diets of this type.

MODIFIED CLEANSING DIET

FIRST TWO DAYS

Fresh fruit only. Any kind of fruit except bananas, rhubarb, plums, gooseberries. The fruit may be eaten raw or cut up into a fruit salad. If fruit salad is made only use a little honey for sweetening, otherwise omit the fruit if it cannot be eaten without further sweetening.

Drinks during these two days may consist of fresh pure (or bottled, unsweetened) fruit or vegetable juices, although it is unlikely that much drink will be required as adequate liquid occurs naturally in the fruit.

THIRD AND FOURTH DAYS

On Rising

Fresh fruit as before, or baked or puréed apples, with raisins.

Between Meals

Fruit juice or savoury drink, e.g., a yeast extract beverage – one teaspoonful in a cup of hot water.

Lunch

Raw combination salad with dried fruit and dressing if desired. No savoury or biscuits are to be taken with the salad at this stage.

Fresh fruit for dessert.

Evening Meal

Raw salad again as for lunch.

Fresh or soaked dried fruit for dessert.

On Retiring

Fruit juice, or savoury drink.

FIFTH TO SEVENTH DAYS

On Rising

Lemon or apple cider vinegar drink (see recipes).

Breakfast

Fresh fruit, or soaked dried prunes or apricots, or baked or stewed or puréed apples. Raisins or wheatgerm may be added to the fruit if desired.

Lunch

Raw combination salad. A portion of milled nuts may now be added, or some wheatgerm may be sprinkled on the salad. Small portion of low-fat or cottage cheese may be taken.

Fresh or dried fruit for dessert.

Evening Meal

Raw salad as before, or mixed vegetable broth, or two or three conservatively cooked vegetables, served with a light egg dish, or a little steamed fish, or a vegetable casserole (see recipes).

On Retiring

Fruit juice or savoury drink as before.

NOTE

The mid-day and evening meals may be transposed if desired. If you are away from home during the day and find it difficult to obtain a meal as described, then you should take fresh fruit, with some nuts and raisins.

This diet may be extended for a further week by continuing to follow the directions for the fifth to seventh days, or you may return to the balanced diet given in the previous chapter.

STRICT CLEANSING DIET

IMPORTANT NOTE

Unless you have been accustomed to a food reform diet, containing a high proportion of fruit and vegetables for some time, you should not attempt to follow this diet without obtaining professional advice from a naturopath.

Whilst it will be of great benefit to the majority of sufferers from asthma and hay fever, some people may not be constitutionally suited to such a diet, and even those who are may experience aggravations, or 'healing crises'. These are often a good sign but you should be guided through them by a practitioner who understands the various stages of recovery. You should also endeavour to rest as much as possible during the first week or two of the diet.

FIRST WEEK

DAYS 1 AND 2

Fast, taking only pure water or fruit or vegetable juices. One tumblerful of juice may be taken four or five times daily according to thirst. Any kind of fresh fruit juice may be used, such as apple, orange, grape, or vegetable juice, such as carrot, celery, or beetroot. The juices should, if possible, be freshly extracted. The vegetable juices can be mixed or combinations may be taken – carrot and apple juice are a good combination for asthma sufferers.

If fresh juices are unobtainable the bottled or canned fruit or vegetable juices may be used, but these should be pure and free of any sweeteners or other additives. Never use 'soft drinks' or squashes, such as the popular brands which have 'added glucose'.

If you prefer a hot drink, one of the brands of pure, concentrated apple juices may be taken with warm water, or a savoury drink may be made using a vegetable

CARROT + APPLE JUICE GOOD FOR
ASTHMA.

concentrate or yeast extract beverage (one teaspoonful in a cup of hot water).

DAYS 3 TO 5

Fresh fruit only. Any kind of fruit except rhubarb or bananas, and certain soft fruits (e.g. plums, gooseberries). Take as much of the fruit as appetite demands, at mealtimes. If preferred fruit can be cut up or grated to make a fruit salad, with a little honey for sweetening if necessary.

For those who, for various reasons, find raw fruit unpalatable or indigestible, it may be puréed or stewed and eaten thus with the addition of some raisins and a little honey for sweetening.

If drinks are required between meals you may take fruit juices or savoury drinks as before, or weak China tea with lemon or a dash of soya milk.

DAYS 6 AND 7

Breakfast

Fresh fruit juice, or lemon and honey drink. Fresh or dried fruit.

Between Meals

One small glassful freshly extracted carrot juice, or mixed fruit or vegetable drink, or warm drink (e.g. weak tea, cereal coffee, etc.).

Lunch

Raw combination salad (see recipes), with dressing, or clear vegetable broth.

Fresh fruit as dessert.

Evening Meal

As for lunch.

SECOND WEEK

Breakfast

Pure fruit juice drink.

Fresh or dried fruit. If made into a fruit salad a little wheatgerm and honey or maple syrup may be added.

For warm drink, if desired, weak China tea or cereal coffee, or herbal tea may be taken (especially peppermint, verbena, or linseed teas).

Between Meals

Fresh cool fruit or vegetable drink as above, or warm drink as above.

Mid-day Meal

Raw salad as above, but you may now add dried fruit and milled nuts and a little cottage or ricotta cheese, or mixed vegetable soup or broth.

Fresh or dried fruit as dessert.

Evening Meal

Raw salad as above, or vegetable soup, or two to three conservatively cooked vegetables in casserole, with a savoury sauce (see recipes) on top.

Fresh fruit or natural fruit jelly or carrageen (seaweed) mould or soya dessert.

THIRD WEEK

Breakfast

As second weeek. You may now have a small portion of goat's milk yogurt with the fruit.

Mid-day Meal

As second week, but you may now take a slice of wholemeal bread, or one or two slices rye biscuit or pumpernickel with the salad or soup. Apply butter or sunflower oil margarine thinly. Use a savoury spread if desired.

Evening Meal

Salad again if desired.

Or savoury protein dish with conservatively cooked vegetables.

FOURTH WEEK

Continuation of fruit and wheatgerm breakfast is desirable. You may now have one or two slices of rye biscuit or wholemeal bread or pumpernickel with sunflower oil margarine or a little butter. Honey should be used rather than other preserves, or you may have a savoury spread.

Of the remaining meals, one should consist entirely of raw salad and fruit, and the other of conservatively cooked vegetables with lean meat, fish, egg, or other savoury dishes. For desserts try to keep to fresh or dried fruit or fruit-based dishes, or biscuits and low-fat cheese.

After completing the four weeks of the strict diet you should return to the balanced diet. It is essential to continue to avoid acid-forming foods or drinks, especially those foods which you are warned against in chapter 3.

During the time that you are on the diet it is important to ensure regular, easy bowel action, and if necessary this may be done during the fasting stage by means of a small warm water enema. At any other time only a herbal bowel regulator should be used. The type which swells in the bowel stimulating normal muscular action of the colon is most suitable. Carry out the physical measures, such as hydrotherapy and exercises during this time to improve eliminative functions, oxygenation and general health.

DIET FOR ACUTE ASTHMA

The acute attack of catarrhal asthma will be characterized by breathing difficulty in association with profuse mucus secretion in the lungs. In the early stages the usual symptomatic treatment may be necessary to relieve the attack but it is also essential to apply stricter dietary measures for several days to enable the body to overcome the congestion and to reduce its exposure to allergenic foods.

At the onset of the catarrhal symptoms or aggravation of wheezing, you should retire to bed and withhold all solid food for at least twenty-four hours. Warm fruit juices or savoury drinks may be taken, or clear vegetable broth. No milky drinks should be given under any circumstances.

57

If the chest becomes tight and breathing becomes difficult, hot fomentations should be used. (Towels soaked in hot water, well wrung out, applied damp to the chest and upper back, and repeated for twenty to thirty minutes, or until some relief is obtained.)

When breathing becomes more normal it would be advisable to keep to vegetable broth or fresh fruit only for a further twenty-four to forty-eight hours before returning to the balanced diet.

FRUIT DAY

When you have started the basic diet it is a good idea to introduce a fruit day. For one day per week eat only fresh fruit at meals and take fruit juices or savoury drinks between meals. Any type of fruit, except rhubarb and bananas, may be taken and you may eat as much as is required to satisfy your appetite.

MILD ELIMINATIVE DIET

This is a diet which can be undertaken by most people with chronic catarrhal asthma from time to time. After being on the balanced diet for at least one or two months this short eliminative diet may be introduced or it may be done whenever there is a sign of catarrh increasing and threatening to cause a return of acute symptoms.

FIRST DAY

Fresh fruit or fruit juices only, as for the fruit day (see above).

SECOND DAY

Breakfast

Fresh fruit or fruit salad with raisins, milled nuts and a little honey or maple syrup to sweeten.

Lunch

Mixed salad prepared as instructed under Basic Diet. Fresh fruit as dessert.

Evening Meal

Mixed salad as before or fresh fruit.

Between Meals

Drinks of weak China tea, coffee substitute made with water and using soya milk, or fruit or savoury drink.

THIRD DAY

Breakfast

As above.

Lunch

As above.

Evening Meal

Salad again, or savoury dish of egg, cheese or fish with conservatively cooked vegetables. Fresh fruit only as dessert.

Then return to the basic diet. This diet can be extended or modified as required. During the early stages of your treatment you will find three days sufficient. If the symptoms seem to get worse when you undertake the diet, slow down the elimination by having a little cooked food, such as a light protein dish with vegetables, or a mixed vegetable soup, or eat one or two slices of wholemeal bread with your salad.

As you progress you may find that you can extend this treatment by staying on the first or second days diet longer, or you may be able to undertake the stricter eliminative diet which follows.

STRICT ELIMINATIVE DIET

This diet should only be undertaken after having followed the basic diet for some weeks, with occasional periods on the mild eliminative diet. It will be of great value to the very catarrhal person who gets repeated attacks of asthma, owing to congestion of the lungs. People who have suffered for many years, or have become dependent on drugs, however, should not undertake the strict diet without the advice of a practitioner who can guide them through the 'healing crises', or aggravations, which may occur.

It is advisable to rest during the early stages of this diet as mild symptoms such as a coated tongue, headache or slight weakness can occur. Such symptoms can be ignored as they will usually pass after a few days when the tissues begin to reduce their toxic overload.

FIRST THREE DAYS

Fruit or fruit juices only. Any kind of fruit except bananas and rhubarb. Eat as much as the appetite demands at each meal. If desired the fruit can be made into a fruit salad and sweetened with a little honey. Fruit juices should be unsweetened and may be taken cold or with hot water.

NEXT THREE DAYS

On Rising

Warm water, lemon juice and honey.

Breakfast

Fresh fruit as before. If fruit salad is taken you may now add some raisins, milled nuts, or pine kernels for flavour. Baked or stewed or *puréed* apple may be taken instead of fresh fruit.

Between Meals

Warm or cold fruit or savoury drink as desired.

Lunch

Large mixed salad containing selection of vegetables in season. (Try to include some raw onions or garlic.) Milled nuts or raisins may be added for flavour. Home-made salad dressing may be used. Take fresh fruit as dessert.

Evening Meal

Salad as for lunch or vegetable broth made with a selection of vegetables in season. Fresh fruit as dessert.

On Retiring

Warm or cold fruit juice drink.

SECOND WEEK

On Rising

Warm lemon and honey drink.

Breakfast

Fresh fruit as fruit salad with raisins and wheatgerm or milled nuts. Baked apple, or stewed, or *puréed* apples with raisins and wheatgerm as alternative.

Between Meals

Drinks as above.

Lunch

Vegetable soup (not tinned). Mixed salad as before. You may now add some milled nuts, cottage or low-fat cheese. 1–2 slices rye biscuit with a little sunflower oil margarine may be taken with the salad if desired. Fresh or dried fruit dish as dessert.

Afternoon

Fruit juice drink.

Evening Meal

Apéritif of apple, carrot or other fresh fruit juice. Light savoury dish (e.g. egg, lean meat, fish, millet, rice or nut dish), with 2–3 conservatively cooked vegetables; or raw mixed salad as for mid-day; or vegetable broth. For dessert, fresh or dried fruit dish flavoured with nuts, pine kernels, maple syrup, etc.

On Retiring

Warm or cold drink as before.

If more convenient the order of the meals may be reversed, that is, the salad meal may be taken in the evening and the cooked meal at mid-day.

At the end of the two weeks continue with the same diet if possible but otherwise return to the balanced diet. You may revert to the second week of the strict diet whenever you feel able to, as this will give a mild degree of relief to any symptoms of catarrhal congestion.

CHAPTER SEVEN

Supplementing Your Diet

In an ideal world our bodies would obtain all the raw materials they require for the maintenance of perfect health from our food and drink. There are a number of reasons why they no longer can: modern agricultural practices have resulted in trace element deficiencies in the soil; fertilizers and pesticides impose an added burden to the body's detoxification mechanism (hence my recommendation to use organically grown produce wherever possible); many food manufacturing processes lead to loss of nutrients; the ability of the body to digest and assimilate even an apparently healthy diet may not always be adequate.

There is, therefore, a need for many people to take nutritional supplements, which should, whenever possible, be prepared from natural ingredients. The science of applied nutrition – the clinical use of vitamins, minerals, and other supplements – has made enormous progress in recent years and one thing that has become clear is the biological superiority of those prepared from natural sources as opposed to chemically synthesized versions.

There are many nutrients which have been found to play a vital role in maintaining the functions of the immune system, protecting against inflammation, reducing excess spasm of muscle fibres, and boosting general energy. There are also some basic herbal preparations which are worth using. I have selected some of the most influential and listed the richest food sources in which they may be found as well as describing supplements. All of these should be readily available from a health food store in a suitable form.

It must be emphasized that food supplements are no substitute for a balanced wholefood diet. In fact, this is essential if they are to do you any good.

VITAMINS

Vitamin A

This vitamin, which occurs naturally in fish, liver, eggs, carrots, oranges, and other yellow fruits, is an important protector of sensitive mucous membranes, such as those of the nasal cavity and sinuses, so it is very useful for hay fever sufferers as well as asthmatics.

The best way to supplement vitamin A is to take Beta Carotene from which it is manufactured by the body. Capsules of 6mg should be taken three times daily with meals.

EAT PLENTY OF: FISH LIVER EGGS + ORANG FRUIT CARROTS I.C. ORANGES ETC.

Vitamin B

This complex of related vitamins (B_1, B_2, B_6, etc.) plays an important role in conjunction with the trace element zinc and some essential fatty acids in the production of anti-inflammatory substances. Rich food sources are whole grains, eggs, brewer's yeast, green leafy vegetables, and liver.

A strong B complex, hypoallergenic formulation may be taken once daily with breakfast.

Vitamin C

Vitamin C is a powerful anti-oxidant which means it reduces the rate of breakdown of body cells, conserves oxygen, prevents inflammation, and helps to strengthen immunity. Research has shown that, where levels are low in the body, supplementing vitamin C can speed up the recovery from colds and other inflammatory illnesses.

Vitamin C is found in green leafy vegetables, cauliflower, broccoli, green peppers, and watercress. It is best to supplement these food sources with the bioflavonoid complex (vitamin C with vitamin P), the state in which nature provides it. 500mg should be taken twice daily. This may be increased to every three hours if you have an attack of asthma or hay fever.

TAKE VIT C. DURING SEVERE ASTHMA ATTACK.

[handwritten: ENOUGH MAGNESIUM IN THE BODY STOPS MUCUS FORMING, NEEDS CALCIUM TO WORK.]

MINERALS AND TRACE ELEMENTS

Some of the basic chemicals upon which our bodies depend for healthy function may be required in increased quantities for a time. The following are the most important.

Magnesium

[handwritten: FOUND IN NUTS, SEAFOOD, SOYA BEANS, GRAINS. GREEN LEAFY VEGETABLES]

Helps to stabilize the mast cells in the mucous membranes so they do not produce so much histamine. Magnesium should dominate calcium with which it works (another reason to avoid cow's milk which contains more calcium than magnesium). Magnesium is found in nuts, seafoods, soya beans, grains, and green leafy vegetables. It is best to supplement it through a mineral compound which will ensure the correct ratio of the various minerals to each other.

Calcium

[handwritten: TOO MUCH ENCOURAGES HISTAMINE RELEASE.]

Calcium is an important mineral in our metabolism and, although it encourages histamine release if too much crosses the cell membranes, it works with other nutrients, including magnesium to prevent this happening.

Legumes, green leafy vegetables, broccoli, nuts, tahini,

and soya milk are among the best food sources of calcium. Dolomite tablets provide calcium and magnesium in a balanced proportion. One or two tablets may be taken three times daily with meals.

Zinc *MAINTAINS CORRECT BLOOD SUGAR LEVELS.*

This is a trace element which is often deficient in the modern diet. It plays a vital role in immunity and in maintenance of correct blood sugar levels. It is present in wholewheat, rye, oats, egg yolk, buckwheat, garlic, and potatoes.

Zinc is available in several forms as a supplement (e.g. Zinc orotate, Zinc gluconate) but it is best to use a multi-mineral supplement unless you have professional guidance as to what is suitable for you.

ESSENTIAL FATTY ACIDS

Essential fatty acids (EFAs) are necessary to transport fat-soluble vitamins, such as A and E, and also play a part in the manufacture of anti-inflammatory prostaglandins. EFAs are polyunsaturated fats, that is they are liquid at room temperature.

The principle sources are sunflower and safflower oils, leafy vegetables, oily fish, nuts, and seeds. You may increase your intake of EFAs with Evening Primrose oil preparations. A suitable dose would be a 500mg capsule twice daily.

HERBAL AND HOMOEOPATHIC MEDICINES

Garlic

The single most important herbal treatment for respiratory disorders is garlic (*Allium sativum.*) Garlic adds flavour to cooking and salads and this is a good way to take it, but, because it is strong on the breath you may prefer to use the tablet form. Tablets made with freeze-dried garlic are the most effective.

Take three or four tablets at night for general prevention and chronic catarrh. In acute situations dose three or four times daily.

Homoeopathic Medicines

These may be obtained from many health food stores or from homoeopathic pharmacies and some chemists. They are natural remedies prepared in infinitesimal doses and the number after the name indicates the degree of the dilution.

ARSENICUM ALBUM 12

Burning, itchy eyes, inflamed throat, streaming, watery mucus, also for the asthmatic who has to lean forward to breathe and is worse between midnight and 2 a.m.

Take a few doses at half-hour intervals or three to four times daily.

KALI CARBONICUM 6

Asthmatic attacks between 3 and 5 a.m. Take every fifteen to thirty minutes.

PULSATILLA 6

Thicker nasal catarrh with old, discoloured mucus. Dose three to four times per day.

SABADILLA 6

Sneezing, itching, frontal headache, sore throat. Take every two or three hours down to three times daily.

CHAPTER EIGHT

Recipes

The following recipes and instructions for preparation of foods are selected with the specific requirements of the asthma and hay fever patient in mind. All the items given may be included in the balanced diet without fear of taking excessive amounts of foods which are harmful in any way. Certain items may, however, have to be avoided when on the stricter diets and these will be indicated in the specific diet.

A selection of basic recipes in the different categories are given. For further variety the reader is referred to some of the many excellent recipe books of vegetarian and food reform dishes now available. When using other recipes bear in mind the limitations imposed on the intake of certain foods during the early stages of your treatment.

SOUPS

It is useful to prepare a vegetable stock which can be used when required. Keep the water in which the vegetables have been cooked and use this in soups and savoury dishes. Savoury spreads like dried brewer's yeast extracts can be used as stock where it is not possible to make some from fresh vegetables. The spread is mixed in hot water in the desired strength.

Mixed Vegetable Soup

Selection of any vegetables in season such as carrots, celery, cabbage, cauliflower, beetroot, leeks, tomatoes, onions, lentils, beans, peas, spinach, potatoes
5 tablespoonsful sunflower seed oil
2 tablespoonsful wholemeal, or soya flour
Sea salt
Herbs to flavour

Sauté chopped onions in sunflower seed oil. Add wholemeal flour (this can be mixed in half portion with soya flour if desired). Dilute with vegetable stock. Add conservatively cooked vegetables and allow to simmer for 10 minutes. Add brewer's yeast extracts, sea salt and herbs to flavour.

Clear Vegetable Broth

Vegetable stock
Sunflower seed oil – 1 dessertspoonful
Yeast extracts etc., to flavour

Sea salt
Parsley, chives or mint

The vegetable stock is heated and poured over the other
ingredients. Allow to simmer for 5 minutes before
serving.

Carrot Soup

2 large carrots
1 onion
1 tablespoonful wholemeal flour
2 oz (50g) sunflower oil margarine (or vegetable oil)
1 teaspoonful thyme or other herbs to flavour
1½ pt (¾ litre) water
Sea salt

Dice carrots; peel and chop onion; sauté in margarine, or
oil, with herbs, for 5 minutes. Stir in flour and add water.
Cook gently for 30 minutes. Season with sea salt, or add
extract to flavour.

Onion Soup

1 tablespoonful sunflower seed or corn oil
2 large onions
5 tablespoonsful wholemeal flour
4 pt (2 litres) of water
Sea salt

Savoury spreads for flavour
Herbs

Sauté onion in vegetable oil until tender. Add and mix flour. Add vegetable stock and sea salt. Cook 30–45 minutes. Sieve if desired, and serve with the addition of savoury spreads for flavour.

SALADS

Combination Salad 1

Half a lettuce
Watercress
Cress
Cucumber
2 tomatoes
Spring onions
2 medium carrots
Mint or parsley
Milled nuts
Cottage cheese

Break lettuce into bowl. Add watercress, sliced cucumber, tomatoes, and grated carrots. Garnish with mint and parsley and add spring onions. Sprinkle milled nuts over the salad. Serve with cottage cheese and sunflower oil or salad dressing.

Combination Salad 2

>Half a head of green cabbage
>2 medium carrots
>2 onions
>Lettuce
>Radishes

Chop finely the cabbage, radishes, carrots. Serve on bed of lettuce with dressing.

Cabbage Salad

>Quarter head of red or white cabbage
>2 onions
>2 medium carrots
>Watercress
>Raisins

Shred cabbage, watercress and carrots and mix with the raisins. Add sliced onions. Serve with salad dressing.

Winter Salad

>Half head of cabbage
>2–3 medium carrots
>Half raw beetroot

Celery
1 green pepper
1 onion
Chicory
Nuts
Raisins
Small portion Cheddar cheese

Chop or dice the cabbage, celery, pepper and onion. Grate the carrots and beetroot. Mix all ingredients together in a bowl and add milled nuts and raisins. Break chicory on top and sprinkle dressing over salad before serving.

Apple and Vegetable Salad

1 apple
Celery stalks
Lettuce leaves or endive
Cucumber
Nuts

Chop the celery, endive and cucumber. Mix in bowl rubbed with garlic cloves. Add apple slices and sprinkle with milled nuts. Serve with salad dressing.

SALAD DRESSINGS

Lemon and Honey Dressing

Corn or sunflower seed oil
Pure lemon juice or apple cider vinegar
1 teaspoonful runny honey
Herbs
Sea salt

Mix 75% corn or sunflower seed oil with 25% lemon juice or cider vinegar, add honey and mix in. Add herbs and sea salt to flavour.

Yogurt Dressing

2–3 tablespoonsful yogurt
Lemon juice
Onion or garlic
Mixed fresh or dried herbs

Add few drops of lemon juice to the yogurt and chopped onion or garlic and whisk thoroughly together with mixed herbs.

Tofu Dressing

Half to whole block tofu (200–300g)
Half cup vegetable oil
1 tablespoon tamari or soya sauce
1 tablespoon tahini
Fresh mint leaves

Place ingredients in a blender or bowl and chop or break in the mint leaves. Blend or whisk to a thick creamy consistency. May also be used as a dip.

SAVOURY DISHES

Savoury Grains

Whole cereal grains such as millet, buckwheat, rye or brown rice may be used as a savoury dish.

Place the grains in a saucepan and just cover with water. Bring to boil, replace lid and allow to simmer for 5–10 minutes, or longer according to the grain. The water should be almost absorbed by the grains. Add grated cheese, chopped onions or mushrooms, nuts or raisins, or flavour with yeast extract if desired. Serve with salads, or as a main dish with 2 or 3 conservatively cooked vegetables.

TRY SOYA BEANS, INSTEAD OF
BUTTERBEANS.

Lentil Savoury

8 oz (225g) lentils
2 large onions
3 tablespoonsful sunflower seed oil or corn oil
5–6 peeled tomatoes
6 oz (175g) grated cheese
1 large can soya beans (or fresh soya beans which have
  been soaked for twenty-four hours in water)

Cook lentils in a little water (just sufficient to cover them)
until the water is absorbed. Place in an ovenproof dish.
Chop onions and sauté in 3 tablespoonsful of vegetable
oil. Add soya beans, tomatoes and onions to the lentils.
Spread grated cheese over top. Bake in moderate oven for
20 minutes or until cheese is browned.

Stuffed Marrow

1 medium sized marrow
2 large onions
Mushrooms
Vegetable oil
1 tablespoonful wholemeal flour
¼ pt (150ml) water
1 egg
4 oz (100g) hazelnuts
4 oz (100g) breadcrumbs
Sea salt
Sage or mint

Peel and chop the onion. Wash and chop mushrooms and sauté both in vegetable oil. Mix in the other ingredients and cook for 2–3 minutes. Add sea salt to taste. Cut marrow in half lengthwise and remove the skin and seeds. Stuff with the nut mixture, and put halves together again, securing if necessary by wrapping in greaseproof paper, or foil. Place marrow in tin to which a little oil has been added. Cook in moderate oven for 45 minutes to 1 hour until marrow is tender. Serve with apple sauce, vegetables or savoury grains.

Mushroom and Tomato Savoury

8 oz (225g) breadcrumbs
8 oz (225g) milled nuts
4 tablespoonsful vegetable oil
8 oz (225g) mushrooms
8 oz (225g) tomatoes
Sea salt
Herbs to flavour

Sauté breadcrumbs and milled nuts in vegetable oil, stirring frequently until crisp. Chop the mushrooms and quarter the tomatoes. Sauté these in vegetable oil for 5 minutes. Place a little oil in an oven-proof dish and fill with alternate layers of the mushroom mixture and the nut mixture, adding a little sea salt to each layer, and herbs if used. Top layer should be nut and breadcrumb mixture. Bake for 30 minutes in a moderate oven. Serve with selection of vegetables.

Baked Soya Bean Savoury

1 lb (450g) soya beans
2 celery stalks
1 tomato
4 pt (2 litres) water
1 onion
1 green pepper
Garlic or onion to flavour
Vegetable oil
Pure lemon juice

If using fresh soya beans, soak overnight in water to which lemon juice has been added, then boil for two hours, or until tender, and pour off excess water. Otherwise use canned soya beans from a health food store. Chop celery, onion, pepper and cut up tomato and mix with soya beans. Bake in hot oven for 24 minutes. Add a little oil and herbs for flavouring before serving.

DESSERTS

Fruit Compote

Dried apricots
Raisins
Other fresh fruit in season

Soak the apricots in ½ pt (275ml) of water overnight with the raisins. Simmer for 15 minutes. Add fresh fruit suitably chopped or grated. Cook for 5 minutes and serve with milled nuts or almond cream. Sweeten with runny honey if desired.

Baked Apple

Large apple
Seedless raisins
2 tablespoonsful milled nuts

Core the apple. Fill the centre with raisins. Place in a baking dish in a little water. Bake for 30 minutes. Serve with milled nuts sprinkled on top, and runny honey to sweeten if desired.

Stuffed Pears

4 pears
Almond cream
1 tablespoonful each of raisins, sliced pineapple, ground walnuts or almonds

Halve pears and scoop out cores. Whip almond cream and fold in with raisins, pineapple and milled nuts and place in centre of fruit. Serve with runny honey or maple syrup as desired.

Orange Wobbles

1 or 2 cupsful of pure orange juice
1 small teaspoonful agar-agar or portion of pre-
    prepared carrageen
Runny honey

Whisk agar-agar into half the orange juice and add the honey. Heat slowly over a gentle heat until the agar-agar is dissolved (do not allow to boil). Add the remaining orange juice and mix. Pour into individual bowls and leave in a cool place to set. Serve with a sprinkling of milled nuts or almond cream.

Apple Purée

2 lb (900g) apples approximately
1 cupful of apple juice or water
Runny honey
Lemon peel or cinnamon
Milled nuts

Prepare apples and cut into pieces and cook in apple juice or a little water until tender. Rub through a sieve or prepare in a liquidizer. Mix in honey and lemon peel or cinnamon. Sprinkle with milled nuts and place under grill to brown before serving.

Muesli

Soak organically grown crushed oats in water overnight. Approximately 2 cupsful of water to 1 cupful of crushed oats will be required.

In the morning add 1 teaspoonful of pure lemon juice and grated apple and any other fresh or dried fruit as desired. The muesli may be served with molasses, fruit juice, wheatgerm, milled nuts, or almond cream. Top with goat's or sheep's milk yogurt.

DRINKS

Savoury Drinks

Savoury drinks may be made with low-sodium brewer's yeast extracts.

1 teaspoonful should be mixed in a cup of hot water.

Cider Vinegar and Molasses

Mix together 1 tablespoonful apple cider vinegar and 1 tablespoonful molasses with warm water.

Lemon and Molasses

Mix together 1 tablespoonful pure lemon juice with 1 tablespoonful of molasses and hot water.

Lemon and Honey

Prepare as above, using runny honey instead of molasses.

Herb Teas

These may be obtained in tisanes from a health food store or the dried herb may be used. If the latter method is used, prepare by pouring boiling water over the herb and allow to steep for 5–10 minutes. In the case of linseed tea, 1 tablespoonful linseed to 1 pt (575ml) of water should be used and this should be boiled for 7–10 minutes and then allowed to steep before straining.

Vegetable Juices

These should be freshly extracted in a juicer whenever possible, otherwise the pure bottled variety may be used, including the lacto-fermented type. Juices may be taken singly or mixed together. Carrot and apple juice are of particular benefit.

Index